HOW TO USE GUASHA

Unlock The Art Of Guasha, A Comprehensive Guide To Traditional Scraping Techniques For Holistic Wellness And Pain Relief

LAMBERT FETTERMAN

DISCLAIMER

The content in this book is offered only for general informative purposes. While every effort has been taken to guarantee the content's accuracy and completeness, the author and publisher accept no responsibility for any mistakes or omissions, or for the results of using the information given herein. The methods, recommendations, and directions in this book are not guaranteed to be appropriate for every person, and readers should exercise caution and seek professional counsel if required before undertaking any of the projects or techniques detailed in this book.

Table of Contents

CHAPTER 1

Introduction To Guasha Therapy

Guasha treatment, a traditional Chinese therapeutic practice, has a centuries-long history. Its name, "Guasha," literally translates to "scraping sand," and refers to the scraping or rubbing action utilized in this treatment.

Origins And History Of Guasha

Guasha's treatment derives from Taoist and folk healing traditions in ancient Chinese medicine. Its roots may be traced back thousands of years, developing within Chinese societies before spreading across

East Asia. Guasha was originally used to relieve pain and heal ailments by scratching the skin with different items such as coins, spoons, or horns.

Principles Behind Guasha Therapy

Guasha's central tenet is the belief in repairing the body's qi (life force) and harmonizing the flow of energy or chi via meridian routes. Practitioners utilize implements made of jade, horn, or porcelain to delicately scrape the skin's surface. This scraping movement is said to liberate stored energy, stagnation, or heat in the body, allowing for increased circulation and stress relief.

Benefits And Applications

Guasha treatment has a wide spectrum of possible advantages, making it an adaptable therapeutic approach. Some of its alleged benefits include:

Pain Relieving:

Guasha is often used to treat muscular aches, joint stiffness, and discomfort. The scraping movement is said to promote blood flow, decrease inflammation, and relieve tension, offering pain relief.

Immune Support and Detoxification:

Guasha is said to help in detoxification by facilitating the clearance of toxins and metabolic waste from the body.

This purifying action is supposed to help the immune system and improve general health.

Circulation Improvement:

The scraping action is said to improve blood circulation by increasing oxygen and nutrient supply to tissues and eliminating metabolic waste products, resulting in greater overall health.

Relaxation and Stress Reduction:

Guasha is also known to help with relaxation, stress reduction, and nervous system calmness. Many people find it relaxing and good for their mental health.

Skin Care:

Guasha is said to improve healthier skin by increasing blood flow and promoting lymphatic drainage, perhaps leading to a brighter complexion.

Guasha treatment has evolved throughout time, with variations across cultures and places, each with its own set of practices and equipment. It has received interest in Western alternative medicine practices in recent years and continues to develop as research investigates its effectiveness and applicability in diverse health scenarios.

While Guasha provides comfort and advantages to many individuals, it is important to approach any alternative medicine with care, particularly if you have underlying health concerns. Before beginning any new therapy, it is best to consult with a certified practitioner or healthcare expert to confirm safety and suitability for specific requirements.

CHAPTER 2

Understanding Tools And Techniques

Different Types Of Guasha Tools

Guasha implements vary in material, shape, and size, with each delivering unique therapeutic advantages. Jade, horn, bone, and even ceramic utensils are traditional alternatives. Modern variants, on the other hand, often use stainless steel or resin for convenience and longevity. Individual tastes and therapeutic requirements dictate the design of these instruments, which might be spoon-like, fish-shaped, or ridged. For Guasha, some practitioners may utilize ordinary things like spoons or specifically specialized massage instruments.

Techniques: Strokes, Pressure, And Angles

Guasha's essence is the application of pressure along with mild scraping strokes over the skin. To minimize friction, the practitioner adds an oil or balm to the region. They use the designated instrument to conduct strokes in a certain direction along the body's meridians or afflicted regions, to stimulate circulation and relieve stress. Depending on the patient's comfort and the issue being treated, the pressure used might vary from light to strong.

The angle and strength of the blows are quite important. The tool is held at an angle to the skin, applying consistent pressure while sliding smoothly. Practitioners often work in a set sequence, ranging from lighter to deeper strokes and focusing on areas of tension or stagnation.

Safety Precautions And Hygiene Practices

Guasha treatment places a premium on safety and sanitation. To avoid the transmission of diseases or skin irritations, practitioners must fully clean their instruments before and after each session. Additionally, to minimize bruising or skin injury, use light pressure and vary procedures according to the individual's tolerance.

Hygiene procedures extend beyond tool upkeep. To keep the skin clean, practitioners should wash it and, if necessary, use disposable coverings or towels. It is also critical to educate patients on the feelings they might anticipate during and after the session to guarantee their comfort and knowledge of the therapeutic process.

Following safety procedures ensures not just a nice experience for the receiver, but also the integrity and efficacy of Guasha treatment.

Understanding the subtleties of equipment, procedures, and safety precautions allows practitioners to maximize Guasha's therapeutic potential, encouraging healing and well-being for their patients.

CHAPTER 3

Exploring Meridian Theory

Guasha is a traditional Chinese medicine technique that includes scraping the skin to enhance circulation and treat different diseases. Understanding the fundamentals of meridian theory is critical to understanding the concepts of Guasha's treatment.

Overview Of Meridians In Traditional Chinese Medicine

Meridians are said to be energy corridors that run through the body, influencing its activities. These TCM pathways link diverse organs, tissues, and systems. They create a complicated network that allows Qi, or life energy, to flow. There are twelve basic meridians, each of which is related to an organ system and carries a certain sort of energy. The Lung meridian, for example, impacts breathing, while the Heart meridian influences circulation.

Corresponding Points For Guasha Therapy

These meridians have acupoints or acupuncture points along their courses. These places are often the target sites for scraping during Guasha. Practitioners target certain places depending on the individual's ailment and the accompanying meridian. For example, scraping along the Lung meridian may be used to treat respiratory problems or pain in other regions.

Connecting Meridian Pathways To Overall Health

TCM believes that when Qi movement inside the meridians is interrupted or sluggish, it may cause sickness or pain. Guasha is said to help clear these channels, encouraging the smooth passage of Qi and restoring bodily equilibrium. Practitioners try to treat imbalances associated with certain organs or systems by hitting specific spots along meridians, providing relief from a variety of health concerns.

Understanding meridian theory enables Guasha practitioners to carefully pick locations for therapy, to restore balance and alleviate particular health conditions. Guasha is used to promote the body's intrinsic healing capacities by correcting blockages in Qi flow along these meridian routes, and it is a holistic approach that sees the body as an integrated whole.

CHAPTER 4

Common Ailments And Guasha Solutions

Addressing Pain Relief With Guasha

Guasha is often used to treat a variety of pain disorders, including muscular pain, joint discomfort, and chronic illnesses such as arthritis. Practitioners use scraping movements on problematic regions to promote blood flow, which aids in lowering inflammation and alleviating pain. This approach also causes endorphins to be released, which work as natural pain relievers.

Guasha For Headaches And Migraines

Guasha may provide relief from headaches and migraines when applied to the head and neck. This technique may help relax stiff muscles, alleviate tension, and promote blood flow by gently scraping certain areas or along meridian routes associated with the head, thereby lessening the intensity and frequency of headaches.

Techniques For Specific Body Areas Or Conditions

Guasha techniques may be adapted to particular body locations or health issues. As an example:

• **Back Pain:** Scraping along the spine or the afflicted region helps relieve back pain by relieving muscle tension and improving circulation.

• **Digestive Issues:** Guasha may help improve gut motility and alleviate pain associated with digestive disorders by treating abdominal locations along digestive meridian pathways.

• **Respiratory Health:** When applied to the chest and upper back, Guasha may aid with congestion relief, deeper breathing, and respiratory health.

The particular strokes, pressure, and regions to concentrate on might vary depending on the ailment being treated and the individual's demands.

Guasha may be used in conjunction with conventional therapies as a non-invasive and frequently successful supplemental therapy. However, before taking Guasha, you should visit a skilled practitioner or healthcare expert, particularly if you have any underlying health disorders or concerns.

Practitioners should have a solid grasp of meridian theory, pressure points, and the right use of the method while investigating Guasha for different conditions to guarantee safe and successful results.

Guasha, like any holistic therapy, should be approached as part of a complete wellness strategy that includes good living choices, food, and exercise for the best health.

Would you want to go further into any area of Guasha treatment or learn more about its applicability for particular conditions?

CHAPTER 5

Facial Guasha And Beauty Applications

Facial Guasha entails applying delicate strokes to the face, neck, and décolletage using a smooth-edged instrument, usually composed of jade or rose quartz. The strokes are intended to stimulate blood flow, enhance lymphatic drainage, and relax face muscles. Techniques vary, but most follow the natural curves of the face and certain meridian points.

Facial Techniques And Benefits

The advantages of faceguasha go beyond looks. Improved blood circulation helps the skin get oxygen and nutrients, producing a healthy shine and perhaps decreasing puffiness. It may also aid in the reduction of fine lines, wrinkles, and dark circles beneath the eyes. It assists in cleansing, inflammation reduction, and congestion relief in the face by activating the lymphatic system.

Skin Rejuvenation And Anti-Aging Effects

Facial Guasha is often praised for its anti-aging properties. Increased blood flow and lymphatic drainage may promote collagen formation and skin suppleness and firmness. It is thought that regular practice reduces the appearance of fine lines and wrinkles, resulting in a more youthful complexion. Furthermore, the decrease in face tension and stress might provide the illusion of being calm and revitalized.

Combining Guasha With Skincare Routines

Many people use Face Guasha in their skincare routines. It's usually done after cleaning and adding a serum or face oil to offer lubrication for the Guasha tool's smoother sliding. Users often begin at the neck and work their way up and out over the face, following precise paths and focusing on regions prone to tension or puffiness.

Other skincare products or practices may be used in conjunction with this approach. For example, adding a moisturizer or mask after face Guasha may improve absorption because of enhanced circulation.

While many supporters believe in the advantages of faceguasha, scientific proof supporting its particular cosmetic claims is currently scarce. Individual outcomes may vary, as with any skincare program, and consistency in practice is frequently what determines efficacy.

Overall, face Guasha provides a comprehensive approach to healthcare, combining ancient procedures with current beauty regimens to promote relaxation, and circulation, and perhaps improve skin health and look.

CHAPTER 6

Integrating Guasha With Wellness

Guasha treatment, which is based on traditional Chinese medicine, has a strong relationship between the body, mind, and general health. Guasha, in essence, uses instruments and procedures to stimulate certain places on the body, therefore balancing the flow of energy along meridian routes. Here's a more in-depth look at combining Guasha with wellness:

Guasha For Stress Relief And Relaxation

Stress Reduction:
Guasha's mild pressure and scraping movements are an amazing way to relieve

tension and stress. Guasha relieves muscle tension by targeting regions linked with stress buildup, such as the shoulders, neck, and back. The treatment promotes relaxation by increasing blood circulation and causing the body to produce endorphins.

Relaxation of the Muscles:

Guasha's scraping method promotes muscular relaxation by increasing blood flow and relaxing tight muscle fibers. This aids in the relief of physical pain caused by stress, such as muscle tightness or stiffness.

Emotional Well-Being And Guasha

Emotional Freedom:
Guasha may have a significant influence on mental well-being in addition to its physical

advantages. The impact of the treatment on meridian points associated with emotions enables for emotional discharge. Some proponents think that releasing stagnant energy inside meridians might aid with emotional management, lessening feelings of worry or dissatisfaction.

The Mind-Body Connection

Guasha stresses the link between physical and emotional experiences. It can affect emotional harmony by fostering balance within the body's energy systems. The practice promotes awareness and relaxation while also deepening one's knowledge of the mind-body link.

Enhancing Overall Wellness Through Regular Practice

Holistic Health:

Regular Guasha treatments promote overall well-being by assisting the body's natural healing mechanisms. Its capacity to improve circulation, ease stress, and correct energy imbalances along meridians promotes general health.

Preventive Medicine:

Regular Guasha treatments are not just reactive to stress or pain, but also preventative in nature. Guasha helps to preserve the body's natural homeostasis by facilitating a balanced flow of energy, hence aiding preventative health measures.

In addition, including Guasha in daily or weekly self-care routines enables people to take ownership of their health. Learning simple Guasha practices enables people to handle tension, discomfort, or emotional distress at their leisure, increasing self-reliance.

Finally, the incorporation of Guasha with health goes beyond bodily alleviation. Its ability to reduce stress, improve emotional balance, and contribute to general well-being highlights its importance as a supplementary activity in cultivating a harmonious mind-body connection.

CHAPTER 7

Advanced Guasha Practices

Guasha treatment, which has its roots in ancient traditional Chinese medicine, has gained popularity for its extraordinary effects in improving well-being and treating a variety of health problems. Let's go into advanced Guasha techniques, seeing how this treatment may be upgraded via creative ways and individualized approaches.

Incorporating Essential Oils Or Herbal Remedies

1. Essential Oils: Combining essential oils with Guasha may boost the therapy's effectiveness. Certain oils have medicinal characteristics that enhance the advantages

of Guasha. Guasha may be used with lavender, peppermint, or eucalyptus oils, which have analgesic and anti-inflammatory qualities.

2. **Herbal Remedies:** Herbs have been utilized in traditional Chinese medicine for millennia. Some practitioners use herbal pastes or liniments before Guasha to enhance the therapeutic power of the treatment. When combined with Guasha, herbs such as ginger, turmeric, or ginseng may improve blood circulation and ease pain.

Advanced Techniques For Experienced Users

1.   Deeper   Pressure: Experienced practitioners may use deeper pressure to address deeper muscle layers or chronic tension, guided by the body's reaction. To prevent pain or bruising, this needs close monitoring and competence.

2. Guasha professionals often tailor their strokes, customizing them to individual illnesses or areas of concern. Different stroke orientations, rhythms, or patterns may more accurately activate meridians, enhancing therapeutic benefits.

3. Advanced practitioners may experiment with specific Guasha instruments made of

materials such as jade, horn, or bone, which may provide distinct advantages or subtle pressure adjustments as compared to standard tools.

Customizing Treatments For Individual Needs

1. Tailored Protocols: Skilled practitioners often create tailored Guasha protocols for clients depending on their health concerns, preferences, or reactions to previous sessions. This tailored strategy promotes maximum efficiency and customer satisfaction.

2. Combination treatments: Guasha may be combined with other complementary treatments such as acupuncture, cupping, or

herbal therapy in a holistic treatment plan aimed to address a wide range of health conditions.

3. Client-Centered Approach: Skilled Guasha practitioners stress communication with clients, carefully listening to their input and changing the therapy as needed. This client-centric approach builds trust and guarantees that sessions are tailored to the client's preferences and expectations.

Guasha's advanced methods combine old approaches with current advances, demonstrating the therapy's versatility and effectiveness in treating a wide range of health issues. Nonetheless, consulting with experienced practitioners is essential for the safe and successful deployment of these modern procedures.

CHAPTER 8

Guasha In Modern Healthcare

Guasha's Role In Complementary Medicine

Guasha, previously a traditional medicinal practice, is now gaining popularity as a supplemental treatment in contemporary medicine. It is becoming more widely accepted in integrative medical practices across the globe. Its essential ideas, which are consistent with holistic healthcare, make it useful in combination with traditional medical therapies. The non-invasive nature of the treatment, as well as its potential advantages, such as pain alleviation and stress reduction, contribute to its popularity.

Inclusion in Holistic Healthcare

Guasha's integrative approach complements a variety of medical fields. Its capacity to increase blood flow, relieve muscular tension, and perhaps enhance the immune system has led to its inclusion in wellness programs, chiropractic treatment, physical therapy, and pain management clinics. The comprehensive emphasis of the treatment, which addresses both physical and mental components, is consistent with the patient-centered approach of contemporary healthcare.

Case Studies And Research Findings

Guasha's effectiveness in treating numerous illnesses has been investigated in recent research and clinical trials. Its benefits on pain management, inflammation reduction, and stress alleviation are often studied in research.

While more rigorous scientific data is required, early results point to a beneficial outcome. Case studies illustrating the beneficial uses of Guasha in the treatment of chronic pain, musculoskeletal diseases, and specific skin ailments support the herb's place in contemporary medicine.

Collaborations With Western Medicine

Collaborations between Guasha treatment and Western medicine are increasingly being explored by healthcare experts. Guasha is often used with conventional therapies to improve results or control negative effects. These partnerships aim to improve patient care by combining the qualities of conventional and new techniques. Interdisciplinary talks and seminars create a greater knowledge of Guasha among healthcare practitioners, creating an atmosphere amenable to its incorporation.

Public Acceptance And Perception

Guasha is gaining popularity as people become more aware of supplementary treatments. However, it is critical to provide scientific evidence and ensure safety standards to bridge the gap between old traditions and modern healthcare standards. Education and awareness programs aim to debunk myths and promote informed decision-making about Guasha's position in the healthcare scene.

Guasha's role in contemporary medicine is evolving as more research is undertaken and cooperation with conventional medicine grows. As the discipline develops, its potential advantages and limits will become more obvious, facilitating its incorporation into a variety of healthcare procedures.

CHAPTER 9

Self-Care And Daily Practices

Guasha is an old therapeutic technique that has recently acquired popularity due to its potential advantages for contemporary well-being. Here's an in-depth look at self-care and everyday rituals in Guasha:

Daily Routines And Self-Treatment Methods

Guasha's simplicity makes it easy to include in regular practices. Developing a regular self-care regimen may provide considerable advantages. Begin by designating a particular time or incorporating it into current self-care practices.

Routine in the Morning

Begin your day with a Guasha session to wake up your body. Light, soft strokes may increase circulation, rejuvenate the mind, and relieve sleep stiffness.

Evening Training

Consider using Guasha as part of your nighttime relaxing ritual. Slow, methodical strokes may help relieve stress from the day, enabling a better night's sleep.

Sessions with a Specific Goal

Determine which parts of the body are often tense or uncomfortable. Make your Guasha practice more focused on these areas, spending more time on them to promote relaxation and relief.

Maintaining Health With Regular Guasha Practices

The key to receiving the full advantages of Guasha is consistency. Regular practice may improve general health by increasing circulation, decreasing muscular tension, and improving lymphatic drainage.

Stress Reduction

Guasha is known to induce a relaxation response in the body. Including it in your regimen may help you manage stress by reducing physical and emotional strain.

Increasing Energy

Consider a brief Guasha treatment to revive and re-energize regions including the back, neck, and shoulders for a rapid energy boost.

Immune Boost

Some practitioners claim that frequent Guasha sessions might help the immune system by improving blood flow and aiding in toxin elimination.

Tips For Integrating Guasha Into Daily Life

Making Guasha a natural part of your regimen entails a few easy steps:

Consistency

Even brief daily sessions might be beneficial. Because consistency is more important than length, emphasize frequent practice.

Adaptability

Guasha is adaptable. Experiment with various strokes, pressures, and equipment to see which ones work best for you.

Mindfulness

With purpose and attention, approach Guasha. This practice has the potential to become a kind of self-care that nourishes both the body and the mind.

Learning and Education

Continue to learn more about Guasha. Books, internet resources, and seminars may help you learn more and improve your practice.

By incorporating Guasha into your everyday life, you may reap a variety of physical and emotional advantages, as well as foster a deeper connection with your body and general well-being. Before beginning a new wellness practice, always seek the advice of a competent practitioner and evaluate any personal health problems.

CHAPTER 10

Building A Guasha Practice

Guasha treatment is a traditional Chinese medicine (TCM)-based therapeutic practice. Its name, "gua" meaning scrape, and "Sha" alluding to the redness typically observed on the skin following treatment, refers to the technique of gently scraping the skin with a smooth-edged instrument, increasing circulation and reducing stress. Let's get started with building a Guasha practice:

Training And Certifications

Entering the professional realm of Guasha often requires extensive training. A variety of courses, seminars, and certifications are offered.

These programs often address not just the practical uses of Guasha, but also its theoretical foundations, such as its history, meridian theory, and methodology.

Aspiring practitioners often begin with basic classes, practicing fundamental strokes and understanding correct instrument usage. Advanced classes dive into the intricacies of many approaches, investigating how to treat particular illnesses, extensively comprehend bodily meridians, and include Guasha in a holistic health practice.

Starting A Professional Guasha Practice

Education and Information:
Guasha proficiency requires not just practical abilities but also a thorough

comprehension of traditional Chinese medicinal concepts. Understanding meridian routes, energy flow (Qi), and the function of Guasha in balancing these systems are all part of this. A broad knowledge foundation helps practitioners to properly explain therapy to clients and adapt treatments.

Equipment and supplies:

It is critical to invest in high-quality Guasha tools. These instruments vary in material and design, enabling practitioners to pick based on their comfort and the requirements of their clients. It is essential for a competent practice to ensure the cleanliness and sanitation of these instruments between sessions.

Creating a Healing Space:

It is critical to create a welcoming atmosphere for customers. This entails creating a clean, calm environment that encourages rest and healing. The whole experience is enhanced by soft lighting, calming music, and a comfy treatment table.

Client Acquisition and Networking:

Development of a customer base requires networking and connection development. Participating in neighborhood events, visiting health fairs, cooperating with other wellness practitioners, and using social media platforms may all assist to raise awareness and attract customers.

Resources And Further Learning Opportunities

Education is essential in any therapeutic process. Staying current with the newest research, methods, and advancements in Guasha treatment may be aided by expanding one's knowledge via books, seminars, or internet resources. There are also options for higher qualifications and specialization in certain areas to meet the demands of individual clients.

Starting a Guasha practice requires a combination of knowledge, enthusiasm, and commitment to holistic health. Continuous study, along with a sympathetic attitude toward the well-being of clients, may develop successful and rewarding work in the field of Guasha treatment.

Conclusion

Guasha is a historic and time-tested holistic healing treatment that has crossed ethnic barriers, bringing a unique approach to health and well-being. As we near the end of our journey through the realm of Guasha treatment, it becomes clear that this ancient technique is more than just traditional medicine, but also a flexible and important instrument in contemporary healthcare.

Journey Retrospection:

Our experience through the many facets of Guasha's treatment has been eye-opening. We started by looking into the beginnings of this ancient technique, discovering its origins, and comprehending the fundamental principles that govern its use. Guasha has shown to be a durable and adaptable healing art from its earliest historical origins to its modern significance.

Techniques and tools:

Understanding the many tools and methods used in Guasha is a critical component of learning the discipline. We looked at a variety of Guasha implements, from classic buffalo horns to contemporary variants made of jade or rose quartz. Understanding the appropriate strokes, pressure, and angles is critical to a good Guasha practice, and we went over the finer points of these methods. Furthermore, we stressed the need to follow safety procedures and maintain excellent cleanliness throughout Guasha sessions.

Meridian Hypothesis:

Guasha's congruence with traditional Chinese medicine's meridian theory is critical to its success. We explored the complex network of meridians, locating matching sites for Guasha treatment and understanding the relationship between meridian routes and general health. Guasha is distinguished as a complete and integrative treatment by its holistic approach to healing, which focuses not only on individual symptoms but also on restoring balance to the whole body.

Guasha in Modern Medicine:

Our investigation expanded to the present environment, where Guasha has found a home in modern healthcare. The usefulness of Guasha in supplementing Western medicine became clear when we analyzed case reports and study data. Collaborations between traditional practices and contemporary healthcare are opening the way for a more comprehensive and all-encompassing approach to patient well-being.

Daily Practices and Self-Care:

A key component of our research is equipping people with self-care information and methods.

We spoke about everyday routines and self-treatment strategies, highlighting Guasha's accessibility for personal well-being. Integrating Guasha into everyday life arose as a practical and long-term method of sustaining health and avoiding imbalances.

Developing a Guasha Practice:

We offered information on training, certificates, and the process of creating a professional Guasha practice for anyone who was motivated to learn more about Guasha. Recognizing the increased interest in alternative medicines, we highlighted resources and further learning opportunities to help people on their path to mastering Guasha.

Embracing an Age-Old Tradition:

Finally, Guasha's treatment enables us to embrace a time-honored practice that transcends nations and generations. Guasha's capacity to integrate old knowledge with current thinking makes it a useful tool in the search for holistic health. As we come to the end of our journey, may the information obtained inspire a seamless integration of Guasha into everyday life, promoting a deep connection between mind, body, and spirit.

THE END

9 798871 498224